The Ten Commandments

Of

Makeup

VALENCIA POURIER

To my Fantastic Four,

Never let anyone tell you that your dream is too big.
If you can dream it, then you CAN do it!!! You were born
with everything you need to be GREAT! I love you!

- Mom

Table of Commandments

#1: Thou shall cleanse thy skin day and night.

#2: Thou shall prepare thy skin for the slay.

#3: Thy face and foundation shall cleave and become one.

#4: Thou shall sprinkle clean water upon thy brushes, and they shall be cleaned from all filthiness.

#5: Thou shall come from among all "evil brow doers" and be ye separated.

#6: Thou shall apply your blush good and acceptable, which is thy reasonable service.

#7: Thou shall let patience go before you and make crooked liner straight.

#8: Thou shall not take the word "blending" in vain.

#9: Thou shall give life and moisture unto thy dry lips.

#10: Thou shall "Set it" and "Forget it."

Commandment #1

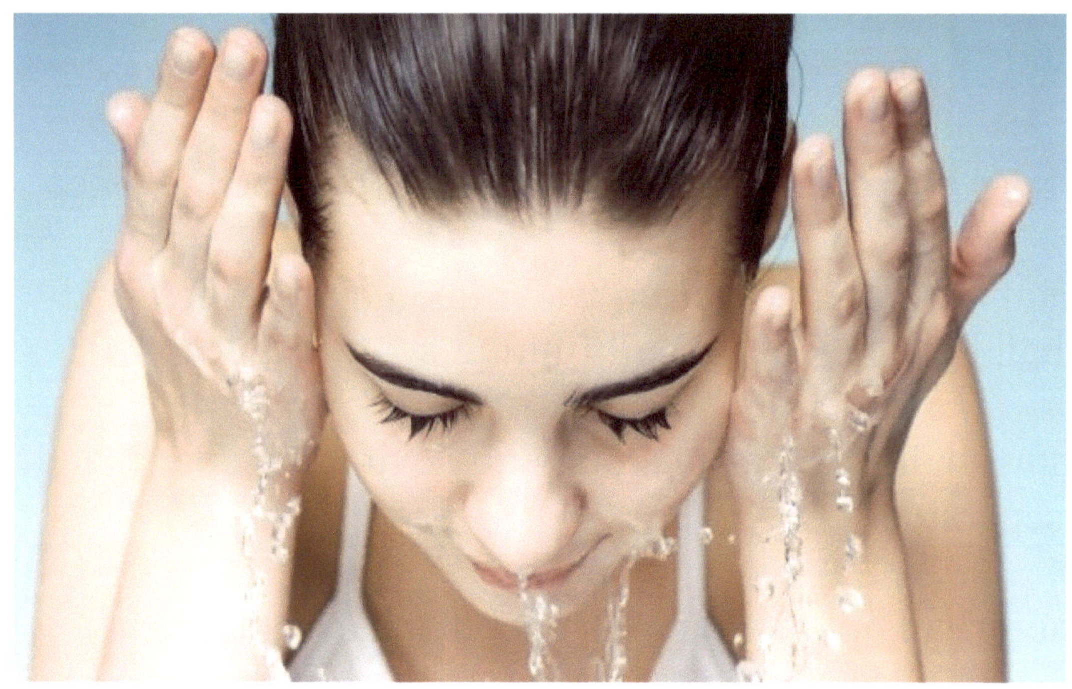

Thou Shall Cleanse Thy Skin Day and Night

*W*e've all heard the saying to "Love the Skin You're In". But what does it mean to truly love your skin? It means taking time to nurture and care for your skin. When it comes to the skin care department, you may find yourself in the twilight zone standing in the middle of a long aisle, filled with skin care products. Searching for the right products can be nothing short of a nightmare if you're not sure what to get. The great news is I'm here to help! You're daily morning skin care routine should consist of a cleanser, toner and a moisturizer with an SPF. These products will differ upon your skin type and your skin needs. Using products that are not tailored for your skin type, may cause the opposite of your desired results. For an example, if you have oily skin, and you're in search of oil-controlling cleansers and etc. You wouldn't reach for products that are made for dry skin. By doing so, you will find that your skin will be more shinier than usual. I call this the Tin-Man effect. (LOL) By reading this you may be asking yourself, "What is my skin type?" Knowing your skin type is essential. Not only for your skin care lineup, but for also choosing the right foundation for your skin. The secret to great looking makeup is to maintain great looking skin. You're never too old or too young to care for your skin. Earlier in this chapter, I mentioned your morning routine. But did you know that you should also have a nightly routine as well? Your nighttime routine may be a bit more tedious, because you will be adding more products. A nighttime regimen should consist of a makeup remover, cleanser, serums or retinols, (for wrinkles, hyper-pigmentation and dullness) eye creams, and a moisturizer to seal it all in. Once you get the hang of it, it will be as easy as 1,2,3! Always remember, what you do for your face, do to your neck also. The skin on your face and neck will thank you later. Great skin doesn't happen by chance, it happens by consistency.

Commandment #2

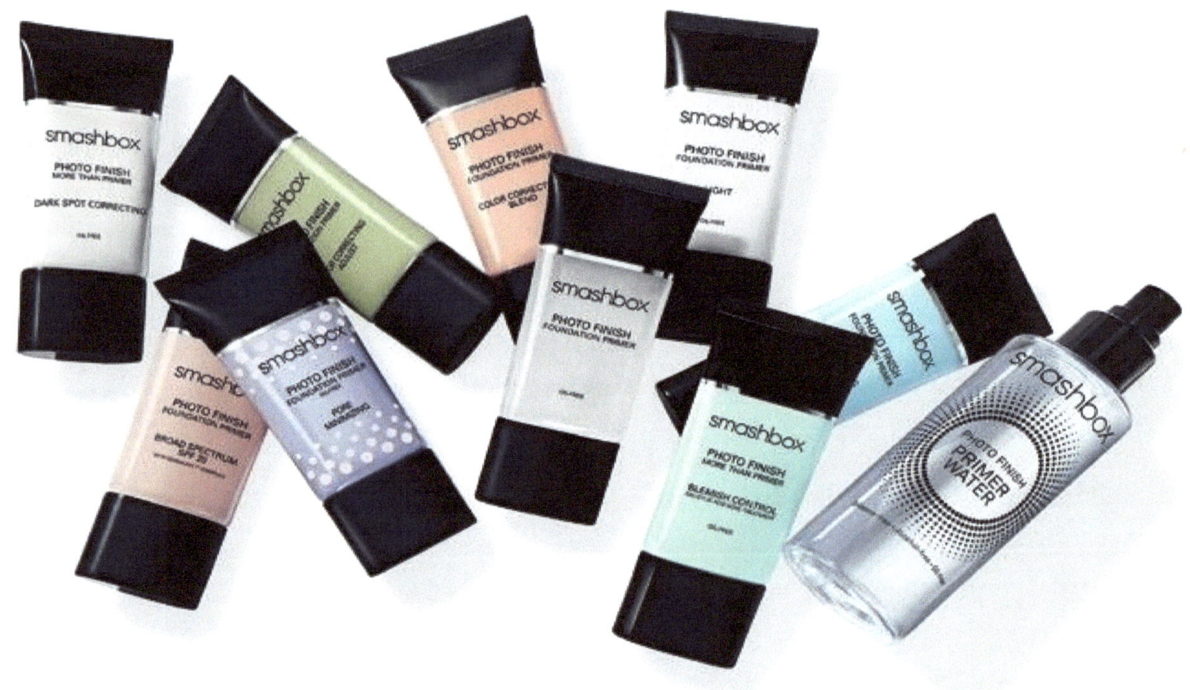

<u>Thou Shall Prepare Thy Skin for the Slay</u>

*S*o now that we've got the skin care out of the way, and your skin is clean, refreshed and renewed. We are now going to prepare the skin for foundation by using a primer. Primer is essential for any foundation, face powder, or eye shadow application. Makeup primer is a product that is used as a base for foundation that allows it go on smoother. your foundation will adhere to the primer and your makeup will last a lot longer than if you were to skip out on using a primer. There's many different types of primers. They're available in cream, powder, gel and liquid form. Primers are also help agents that assist in smoothing fine lines, wrinkles, and minimize the appearance of rather large pores. In the previous chapter, we discussed the importance of knowing your skin type. No matter what your skin type or concern, there is a primer just for you. In addition to the benefits already listed. There are many more that include softer skin, oil control, (and in some primers) a highlighted glow. There are also primers on the market that will color correct and treat skin conditions such as acne, rosacea and eczema. However, if you do have a skin condition, always get advice from your dermatologist. They can recommend products that will work best for you. So now that you have primed your face, don't forget to prime your eyelids. Priming your lids are just as important as priming your face. When you use an eye primer, you are taking necessary precautions to prevent your eye shadow from creasing, and from having "raccoon eyes" at the end of the day. If you are someone who has oily eyelids, you definitely don't want to skip this step. Some of the best eye primers to use is the Urban Decay Primer Potion and the MAC Paint Pot. These primers are considered to be the "Holy Grail" of all eye shadow primers. Makeup artists around the world swear by these products.

They have a blend-able texture that's easy to apply. They are available in different shades and finishes. No matter what eye shadow you use, rather its matte, sparkly or loose powder, you can be sure that your eye shadow will stay! You have many primers to choose from. Whats your pleasure? If you don't have a primer, hurry and get one. Every foundation and eye shadow needs a mate.

Commandment #3

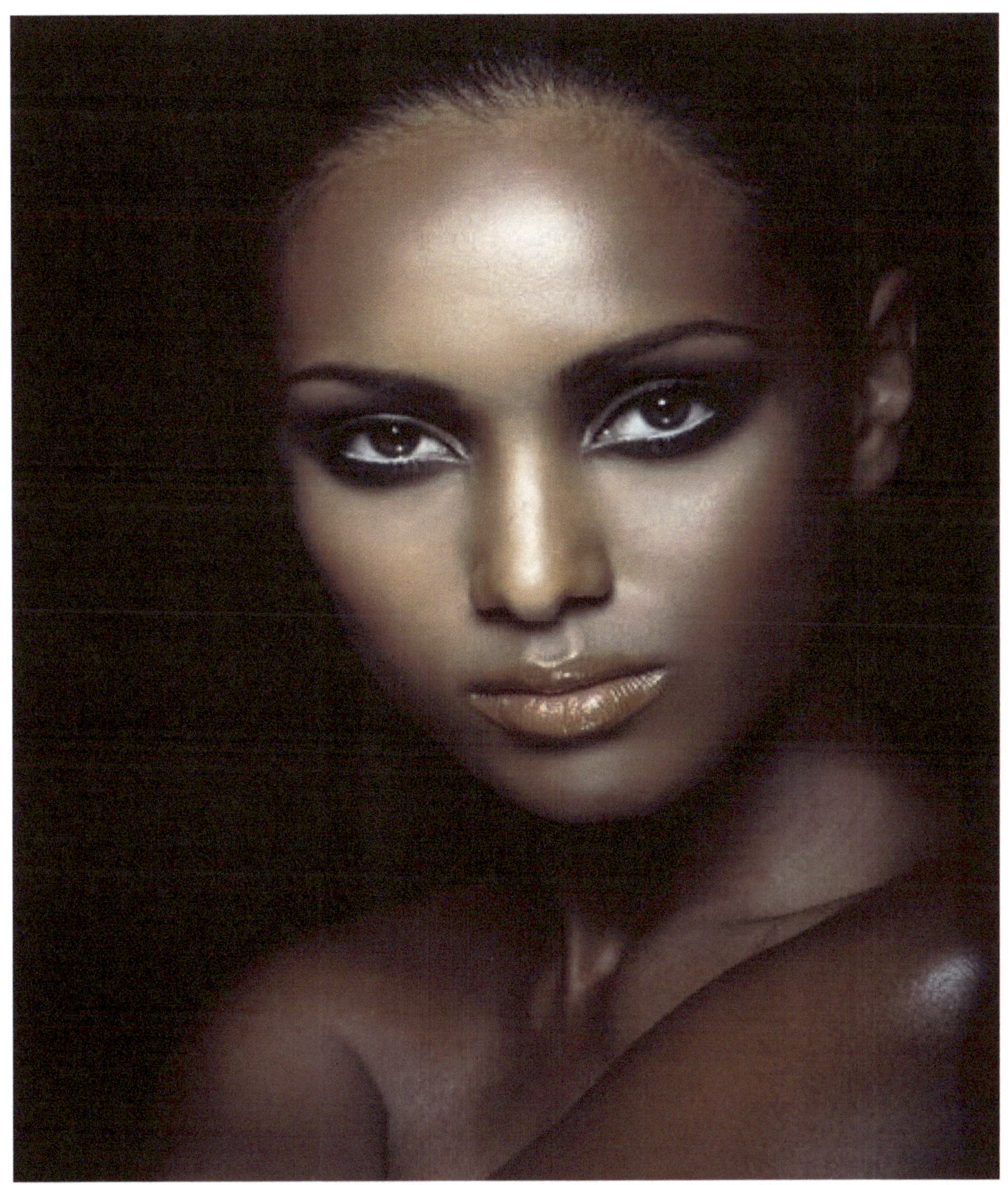

Thy Face and Foundation Shall Cleave and Become One

*H*ave you ever been in public and seen someone with such badly matched foundation, that it appears as if they were wearing a mask? I most certainly have, and unfortunately its a very common offense among foundation wearers. When it comes to matching your skin to a foundation, it can be very tricky. The first step to getting your perfect shade is to know your undertones. A simple way to learn your undertones is by looking at your veins in your wrist. If your veins are yellow or a greenish color, you have warm undertones. If your veins appear to be a mix of green and blue or purple than you have cool undertones. Once you find your correct undertone, you can now find your perfect match. Keep in mind that your foundation should practically "disappear" into your skin. You shouldn't be able to tell where it starts and where it ends. If you're still not sure, then visit your local makeup counter. The makeup counter will have a wide variety of shades and formulas. Someone there will be able to assist you in finding your perfect match. The best way to match your foundation is to do a couple of swatches along the jawline. Whichever shade blends well and disappears into your skin is your correct match. Once you've established your shade you should apply it over your entire face so you can see the fullness of the shade and how it feels on your skin. I'm sure that some of you may be wondering, "How do I choose a drug store foundation"? Choosing a drug store foundation and actually have it match can be a frustrating mission. Especially since there's no testers to swatch or experts available to properly match you. The first step is to "compare". When you pick up a couple shades, and hold them side by side, you will be able to distinguish which shade is warmer and cooler. To be on the safe side, I recommend getting two different colors. Get one that appears closest to your skin complexion, and one that appears a shade darker. In some cases you may need to mix a couple shades to get your perfect match. It may be a difficult task, but don't give up! There's a shade out there just for you.

Commandment #4

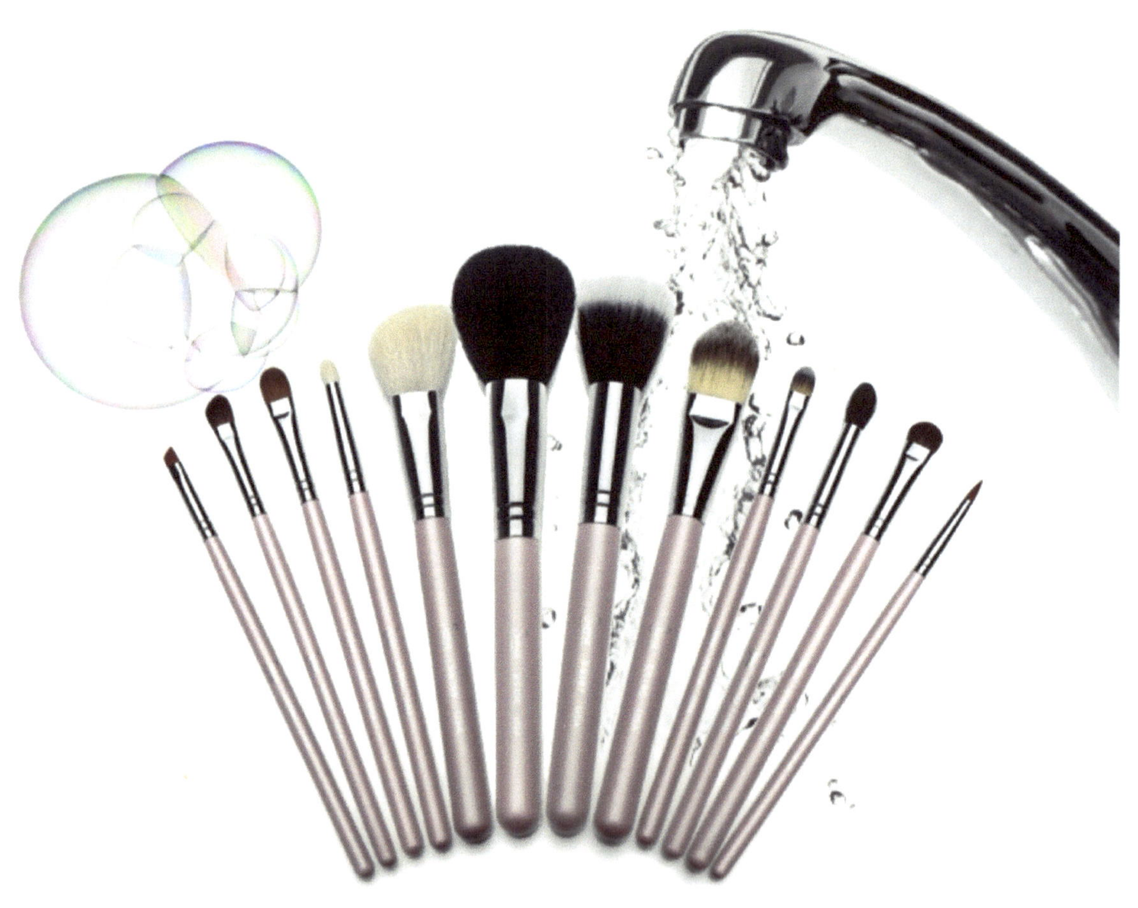

Thou Shall Sprinkle Clean Water Upon Thy Makeup Brushes, and They Shall Be Clean from all Filthiness.

*I*f you have ever visited a makeup counter, and have inquired about, or purchased makeup bushes. Then you probably know that makeup brushes can be quite expensive depending on the brand. I'd like to look at makeup brushes as an investment. And of course, as any other investment, you want to see its maximum return. The best way to do that is to do that is to get a cleansing routine for your brushes. Now you're probably wondering " Why should clean my brushes, if they're for my personal use?" Here are 6 key reasons on why you should clean your brushes:

. Dirt and Debris
. Dead Skin Cells
. Old Makeup
. Oils from Skin and Makeup
. Bacteria
. Changes the Color of Your Makeup

   Not cleaning your makeup brushes, will cause your brushes to get so caked up with old makeup that the bristles can become hard and rough and cause the skin to be irritated. In some cases, may even cause acne. Using dirty brushes will affect the way your makeup applies. Getting flawless makeup is not just achieved by technique, but by clean brushes.

Commandment #5

NO

NO

NO

NO

YES!

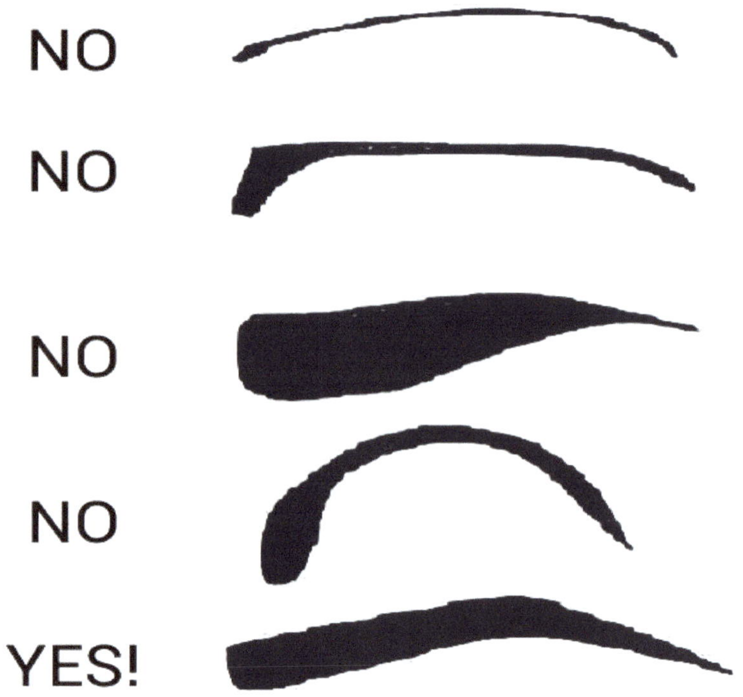

Thou Shall Come from Among Evil Brow Doers and Be Ye Separated.

*W*hen it comes to subject of eyebrows, it may cause a bit of a controversy. With so many products on the market, it can be hard to know where to start. The first step to a perfect brow is to start fresh with a clean brow. Visiting a brow professional will work in your favor. The expert will "clean up" your brows by removing any hair that's not needed in the shape of your brows. Depending on how long your brows grow, your brow tech may even trim your brows. By getting your brows cleaned up, you would be able to see the natural shape of your brow. This will make filling in your brows so much easier. Always remember that the beginning of your brows (AKA the Head) should line up with your nostrils. To fill in your brows, you want to use a powder, pomade or pencil that matches your hair color. Before you fill in your brows, take a spoolie (similar to a mascara wand) and brush your brows in an upward motion. Brushing your brows will allow you too see any sparse areas that need to be filled. For a sharp, dramatic look, add a little product to the tail of the brow to extend it out a bit. But careful, you don't want to extend them too far out. After you fill in the brow take your spoolie and brush the product through your brows to ensure that the product is well blended and your brows are laid. To seal the deal, use a brow gel to help lay your brows down. For an extra pop, you can add concealer that's a couple of shades lighter than your skin tone, under the brow. Not only will it give the brow a more defined look, but it also adds highlight to the brow bone. But make sure that your concealer is well blended. Then you're done!

Commandment #6

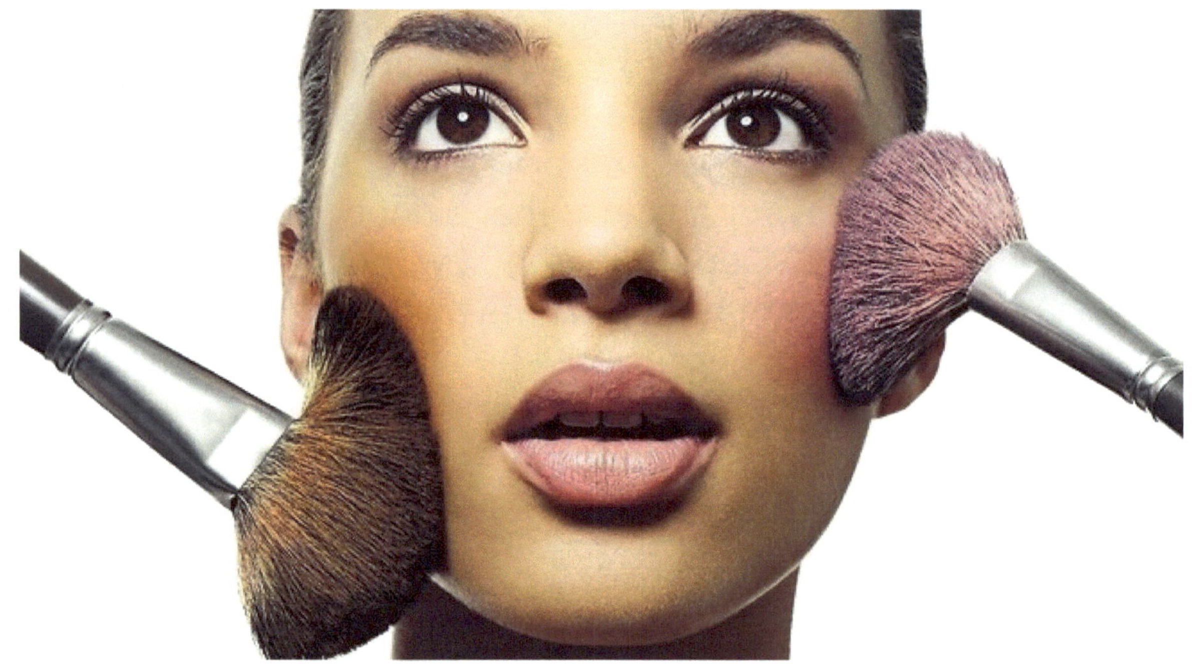

Thou Shall Apply Thy Blush Good and Acceptable, Which is Thy Reasonable Service

*W*here to apply your blush depends on your face shape. Your face shape may be a heart, long, oval, triangle, or round shaped. The eyes of others will draw directly to wherever you apply your blush. So be sure you're applying it in the correct spots. The look of misplaced blush will definitely affect your entire makeup look. Another thing that's really important to remember when applying blush is to make sure you are using the correct blush shades for your skin tone. Unfortunately, blush isn't a one shade fits all product. Using the right shades will not only enhance your makeup, but flatter your complexion. For an example, if you're a woman on the paler side, then you should choose shades that range from light pink to peach to add that perfect flush of color. If you're in the deeper skin tone range, shades like bright peach, apricot and cranberry will give your skin a gorgeous and ethereal glow that will cause heads to turn. When applying blush always remember to use a light hand. After dipping your blush or angled brush in the blush, be sure to tap your brush a couple times to remove excess product. Apply a little at a time. This will prevent you from having the traits of a clown. When applying your blush, be sure to blend, blend, blend! Your blush should blend seamlessly into the skin. If you were a bit heavy-handed and applied too much blush, don't get discouraged. Your makeup isn't ruined. By using a clean brush and sweeping outwards you will buff away some of the excess blush. If that doesn't work and your blush still looks too strong, take a clean brush and use a little bit of translucent powder and apply it on top of the blush. That will diffuse and tone down the pigment in your blush. Sometimes blush can be a little time consuming if you go overboard. But remember, "It's better to arrive late, than ugly".

Commandment #7

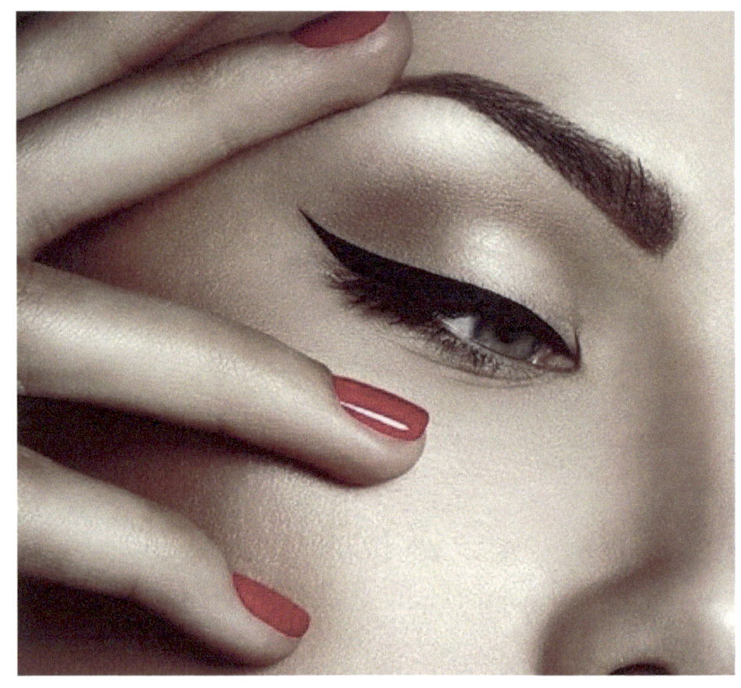

Thou Shall let Patience go Before You, and Make Crooked Liner Straight

*T*here's nothing more frustrating then when you can't seem to get your eyeliner right. The more you add to try and fix it, the more ridiculous you began to look. Don't worry, you're definitely not by yourself. I know the struggle of uncooperative eyeliner. Here are a few tips that will help you win the battle against eyeliner. The first step is patience. Don't rush. Instead of going across your lid in one swipe, draw your line in small strokes or draw dashes across your lid. Then connect the dashes to make one line. Doing so will assist you in keeping a steady hand and will allow you more control over the product. When applying your liner, avoid pulling and tugging the skin around your eyes. Doing so will cause your eyeliner to go on uneven. If you apply your eyeliner and you see areas that are crooked or need to be cleaned up, all is not lost. You can take a q-tip or a thin makeup brush with a primer or concealer to clean up crooked lines or smudges. There's so many eyeliners on the market. Discover which one works best for you and is easier to use. Don't let your eyeliner control you! You have the power to control your eyeliner. Take a deep breath and take your time. You're on your way to being and eyeliner pro.

Commandment #8

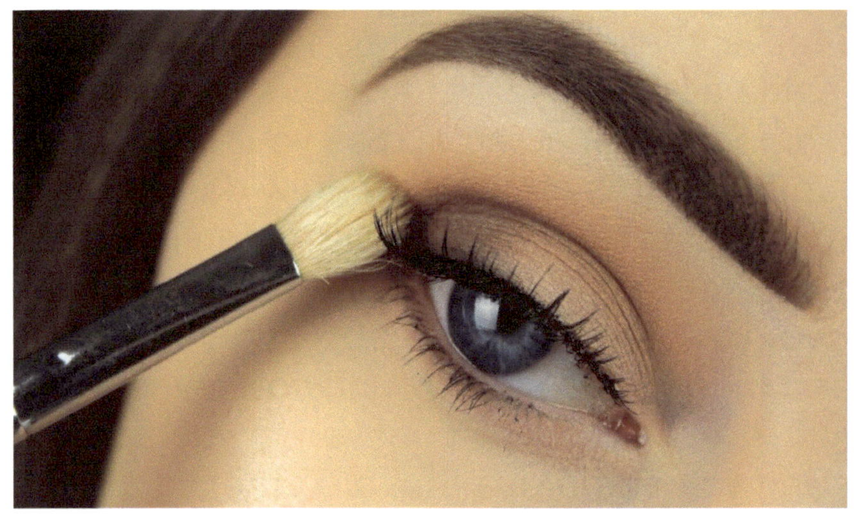

Thou Shall Not Take the Word "Blending" In Vain.

*W*hen it comes to the application of eye shadow, it can become a headache if you're not sure how to use it. Even though Beyonce has tried to convince us that "We Woke Up Like This" the truth of the matter is that we do not. Having a fierce and slayed smokey eye requires work and tedious blending. The purpose of blending is to ensure there is a smooth gradient of colors with no skips, lines or patchiness. If you are properly blending, you can easily wear than one color on your lids at one time. If you're not sure how its done, don't worry. I'm going to give you some blending 101 so you can slay your next smokey eye. The first step is to know which direction you want to go in. Always start blending with your transition color. That is the first color that you place in the crease. Your transition shade is the eye shadow that will help "merge" the other colors together and adds depth to your eye look. To apply your transition shade use a blending brush, then go in windshield wiper and circular motions to blend out the color. Depending on the desired look, always work with the lightest shade first. Sometimes by placing the darker colors first, the pigment can be intense and make your shadow look muddy if you apply too much and its not properly blended. And of course, like anything else to tools and supplies matter. Having a Ride-or-Die blending blush is key to slaying your eye shadow. Some of my favorites are the #224 and #217 by MAC and the Morphe M505. Those brushes blend product effortlessly and give an airbrushed look to your shadow. Following these few steps, will have you blending like a pro. Let's stop eye cruelty and make blending our cardio.

Commandment #9

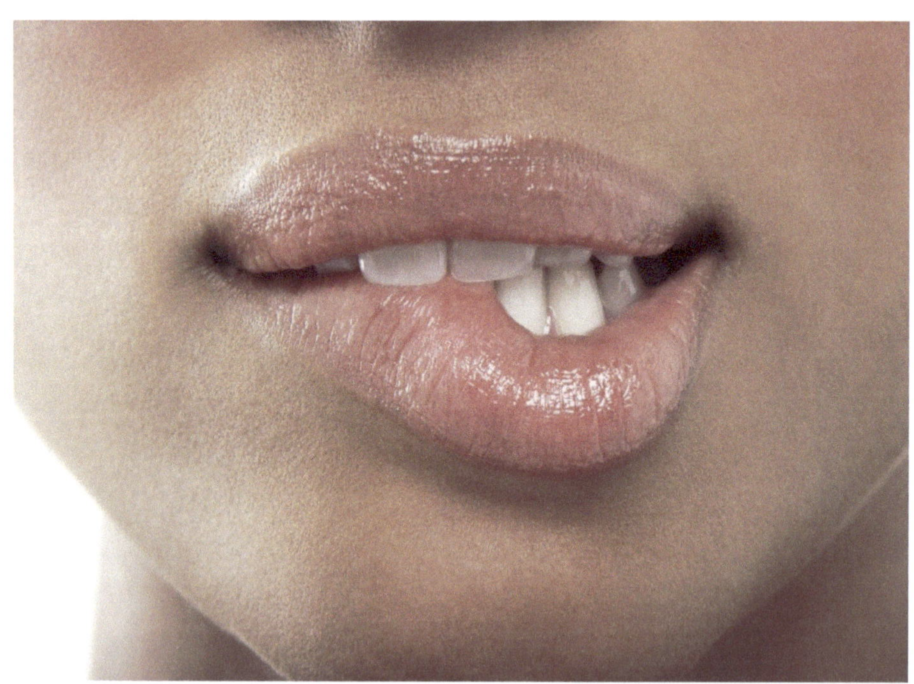

Thou Shall Give Life and Moisture To Thy Dry Lips

Can these dry lips live? O Lord God, You know. The answer is yes! There is hope, revival and restoration for dry cracked lips. Having moisturized lips is more important than you think. Besides the obvious benefit of lip balm, which is to prevent your lips from being cracked and dry, a good lip balm serves other purposes. Did you know that having a well hydrated pout will make you appear younger. When your lips are hydrated, they look more healthy, fuller and it minimizes lines and wrinkles that are on and around the lips. Another benefit is that your lipstick will look 10x's better on hydrated vs. lips that are chapped beyond belief. If you're a bright lipstick lover, having dry lips will cause your lipstick to rest in the cracks and will accentuate the dryness in your lips. To get that perfect pout you should moisturize everyday and exfoliate at least 2x's a week. Exfoliation is just as important as lip balm and partner together for the wellness of your lips. Just as we exfoliate our face, we should exfoliate our lips also. Exfoliating will remove all dead skin cells and allow new collagen in our lips to be formed. Which in turn will make our lips appear fuller and cause the blood to circulate in our lips. There's many exfoliators to choose from, but my go-to is the Tarte Maracuja Lip Exfoliant. It not only removes the dull, dry skin, but it restores the moisture with Maracuja Oil. Find an exfoliator and lip balm combo that fits your needs. Let's show our lips some love!

Commandment #10

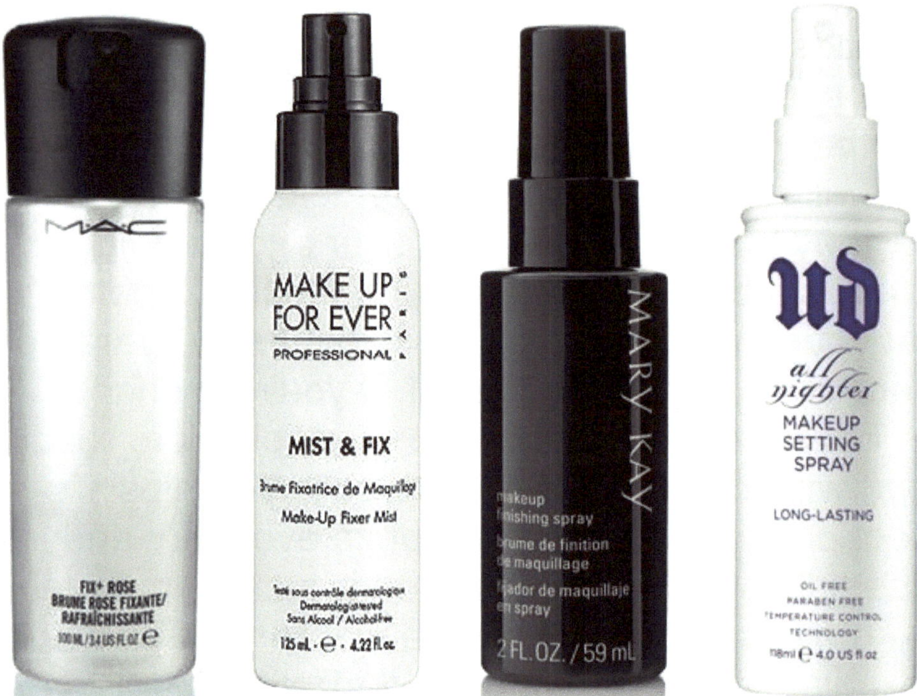

Thou Shall Set It and Forget It!

*S*o, now that you've got your makeup on. You've admired your slayage in the mirror and gave yourself 3 snaps in a "Z" formation. You are now ready to go and Slay your Runway. But wait! You forgot something, you didn't set your makeup. Just like any other expensive art piece, you want to showcase it as well as protect it. You're face is no different. Once you've completed your makeup, you need to use a setting spray. Using a setting spray is what holds it all together. Setting spray is designed to prevent all makeup including foundation, eye shadow, and lipstick from fading, smudging or creasing. Depending on which kind you get, some setting sprays can even help with hydration. If your skin is oily, they have sprays that can assist in oil control and prevent "makeup meltdowns" caused by excessive oil on the face. Setting sprays can be your makeup's best friend, but if used improperly it can cause more harm than good. When applying, hold the bottle about 6-8 inches away from your face. Spraying it too close can cause your makeup to run. After you've sprayed your face, allow it to naturally air dry. Don't try to blend or rub it in. It will cause your makeup to smudge. Once your face dries, your face is complete. Ready, "SET", go!

May your foundation match your neck,
Concealer be creaseless,
And your winged eyeliner be sharp enough to kill.

-Amen-

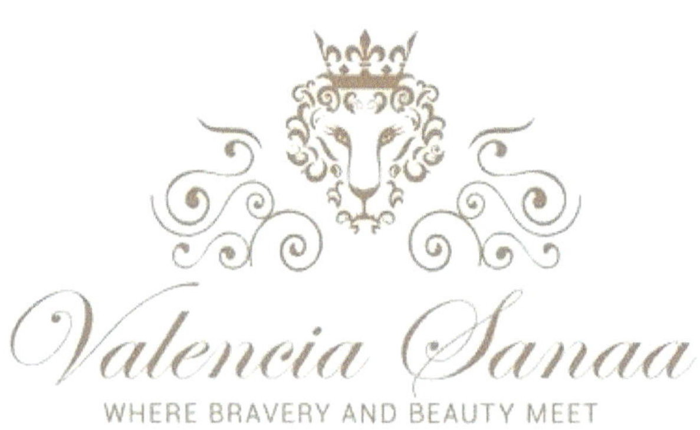